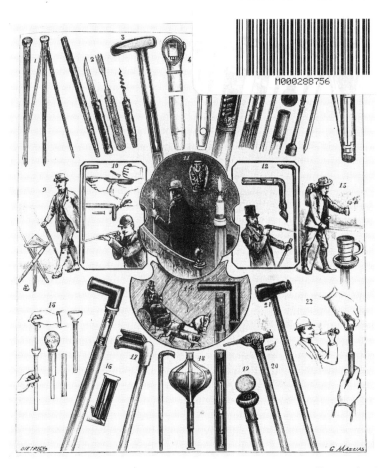

The French magazine 'La Nature' of May 1894 illustrated various gadget walking sticks: 1, camera tripod; 2, fork, knife and corkscrew; 3, mineralogist's cane; 4, still camera; 5, toilet kit; 6, watercolourist's cane; 7, inkstand and penholder; 8 and 9, seats; 10, gun cane; 11, candle; 12, revolver; 13, drinking mug; 14, hand warmer; 15, cigarette-making machine; 16, surgical instruments; 17, snuffbox; 18, Venetian lamp; 19, matchsafe; 20, cigar holder; 21, opera glass; 22, tinder lighter.

WALKING STICKS

Catherine Dike

Shire Publications Ltd

CONTENTS

Introduction 3

History 5

Decorative walking sticks 6

Gadget sticks 17

Further reading 31

Places to visit 32

Published in 1999 by Shire Publications Ltd, Cromwell House, Church Street, Princes Risborough, Buckinghamshire HP27 9AA, UK. Website: www.shirebooks.co.uk

Copyright © 1990 by Catherine Dike. First published 1990; reprinted 1992, 1996 and 1999. Shire Album 256. ISBN 0 7478 0079 0.

Printed in Great Britain by CIT Printing Services Ltd, Press Buildings, Merlins Bridge, Haverfordwest, Pembrokeshire SA61 1XF.

British Library Cataloguing in Publication Data: Dike, Catherine. Walking Sticks. 1. Wooden walking sticks. I. Title. 680. ISBN 0-7478-0079-0.

Collection and photography by Catherine Dike.

Cover: A small selection of the great variety of canes which a collector can find.

A gun case signed 'John Blisset, 323 Holborn, London' which contains an air-gun cane with one grooved barrel. The other cane has interchangeable barrels (one smooth, one grooved). The pump bears the same name as the gun cane.

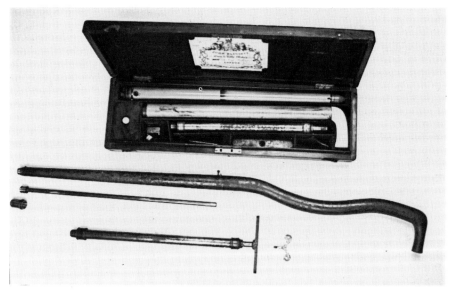

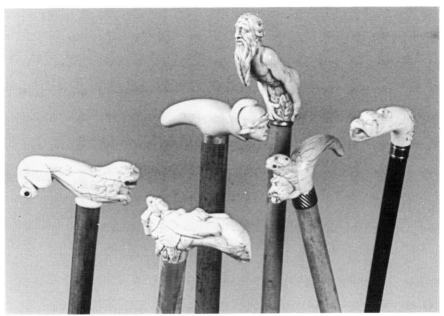

Eighteenth-century ivory handles are more often found in museums than in private collections.

INTRODUCTION

Walking sticks were part of the fashion, style and customs of our forefathers, especially during the eighteenth and nineteenth centuries, and have recently become much sought after by collectors. One cannot but be amazed by the great diversity they show — in their history, their purpose, their artistic value and their role in the worlds of fashion, science, sport and armoury. Because of the great variety of materials used — silver, crystal, porcelain, ivory — and the abundance of gadgets and themes — musical instruments, watches, primitive and folk art — the collecting of walking sticks overlaps into other collections.

Today walking sticks are rarely used as an accessory of fashionable dress. Primarily they are regarded as orthopaedic aids and support for the elderly. The walking sticks in this book would not serve that purpose. They were not intended to be leaned on. They were not physical supports and crutches. On the other hand they were psychological supports. They were an extension of the arm. They gave the owner an elegant air. He could swagger and swing his walking stick to the rhythm of his pace. He could pose and posture with it. He could challenge, defy, flirt and command. In those days one did not carry a walking stick or use a walking stick, one 'wore' a walking stick.

THE TERMS

Before turning to the history of walking sticks, a short description and definition of terms will be useful. The *handle*, by which the stick is held, can be of various shapes and materials. A *knob* is a simple round or cylindrical decoration. A handle is T-shaped and takes a large variety of forms. The *shaft* is the straight part of the stick. If the shaft and handle are of different materials, they are joined by a *band* or a *collar* which serves to hide the joint. Some canes have *wrist cords* that pass through an eyelet under the

3

handle. A *ferrule* or tip, usually of metal, protects the end of the stick. To match the handle, it may also be made of any one of several materials, including ivory, horn, silver or gold. Before roads were tarred the ferrule was 3 to 4 inches (75-100 mm) long in order to protect the wood of the stick from mud.

In Great Britain the term *walking stick* is primarily used, whereas in the United States the word *cane* is used more often. Both terms are used in this text synonymously. The term *stick* has a more rustic and earlier connotation. A collector of walking sticks is known as an *ambulist*.

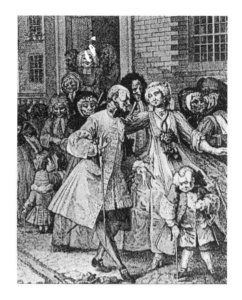

Right: 'Noon' by William Hogarth (1697-1764) shows how the walking sticks of the eighteenth century were 'worn', often hung on the wrist.

Below: A selection of decorative canes: (from the left) a stylised bird in silver, a pewter face on a snakeskin, a silver elephant, three ivory horses, a dog carved from an antler, an Indian's face carved in petrified wood, a plastic lady with a fan, a silver devil chasing a lady up the shaft, an Art Nouveau bronze lady, an ivory greyhound, a wild-boar tusk, a Chinese netsuke knob, a silver Tiffany eagle, an ivory Atlas, a metal devil's face with a natural horn. In front, a crook handle with segments of ivory and horn, and a small ivory dog's head (a child's walking stick).

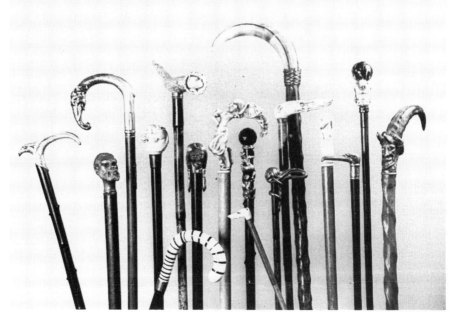

4

HISTORY

Quite probably, the first man who had difficulty in standing up straight took a stick — a branch from a tree — to help stabilise himself. That same branch became his first weapon. As the centuries passed, man added to the basic stick a stone, then a point and finally a hatchet. The stronger the man, the heavier the stick. The largest and perhaps the most beautiful of a community's sticks would have belonged to the local chief. Even very early sticks were decorated, often with carved emblems pertaining to the tribe, its gods, its fears, its fallen enemies. Writers on prehistory often refer to staffs with carved antler horns or mammoth ivory as *chief's batons*.

The first mention of a stick in our civilisation occurs in the book of Genesis: Cain killed his brother, Abel, with a stick. Later Moses led his followers with a stick, and various leaders are often referred to as having an imposing staff. In the New Testament the stick became more an instrument of protection — a shepherd's staff which later became a tau cross and then a bishop's crosier.

In ancient Egypt a stick was an object of prime importance. Everyone used one, but they were not all of the same shape. The form depended upon whether the owner was a shepherd, a merchant, a high dignitary, a priest, a Pharaoh, or even a god! The stick was a necessity not only in life, but also in death. It was placed in the coffin beside the mummy to help and protect the deceased on his travels. Some tombs even contained a great number of sticks — most notably that of Tutankhamun, where no less than 132 sticks were found.

Sticks and staves are found in most ancient civilisations, often elaborately decorated, with various meanings and all kinds of uses. The middle ages were dominated by the church and there we find the tau crosses and bishop's crosiers. No pilgrim would be without his stick. Some, the forerunners of later gadget sticks, contained useful hiding places for money, precious stones and secret weapons. It has even been suggested that the first silk-moth eggs were smuggled out of China hidden inside a pilgrim's cane.

European kings knew the value of a cane. Henry VIII is seen in portraits with his hand resting on a cane. It conveyed authority as well as dignity. The inventory drawn up at his death described an amazing number of walking sticks, some of which could even be called 'gadget sticks'. A famous portrait of Charles I by van Dyck shows him in a very regal pose with his right hand resting on a walking stick.

Louis XIV of France 'wore' high canes and the court followed suit, although they were not allowed to appear before the king with a cane. Despite its aristocratic associations, not even the French Revolution was able to banish the cane. It changed shape somewhat but continued its long life well into the nineteenth century. Another king who 'wore' a walking stick, even on horseback, was Frederick the Great of Prussia. The knobs and handles on many of his were created by the leading jewellers of the day.

With industrialisation in the nineteenth century handles began to be manufactured by the hundreds of thousands. Millions of canes were imported from China. Scores of shops that specialised in both walking sticks and umbrellas flourished. In all the great cities of Europe and the United States models were designed and created by the world's leading silversmiths. Some of the best known in America were crafted by Gorham and Tiffany.

Today's collections fall into two categories: decorative canes and gadget sticks. Both types were used as walking companions in the country, and in town too, but there they were considered a part of fashionable attire.

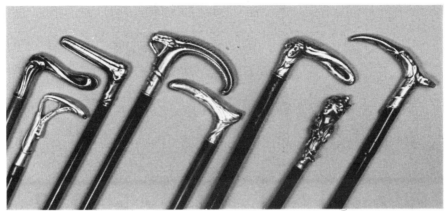

A selection of Art Nouveau metal handles.

DECORATIVE WALKING STICKS

The decorative walking sticks that are found today are mainly those of the late nineteenth century and up to about 1920, when the cane as a fashion accessory began to disappear, followed shortly by spats, waistcoats, capes, *et cetera*.

Silver handles were manufactured by the thousands, and in countless different shapes. Therefore they still form an attractive base to any collection. One can find simple silver knobs, more elaborate animal figures, even the human figure in a reclining position. The Art Nouveau style inspired some of the most creative designs of the period.

Ivory handles, like those in silver, were shaped into a multitude of subjects, in any one of which the collector may specialise. Practically every type of animal has been represented: dogs, horses, tigers, elephants, bats, insects, butterflies, *et cetera*. Flowers and vegetables also made popular knobs. Anything which was a decorative element for other objects in silver and ivory was also used on walking sticks. They were an element of fashion and the favoured embellishment of a cane changed as quickly as a hem line does today.

Porcelain handles of the nineteenth century were mainly made from moulds of the eighteenth century. They are best collected for themselves, that is without a shaft, because on a shaft they tend to knock against one another and can be easily damaged. Displayed on a shelf they make a handsome collection.

Wooden handles were often carved by pipe makers and were later attached to a stick. Folk-art canes were usually whittled by shepherds, prisoners of war and others with time to occupy in winter. The subjects were carved individually by hand. Today, in the United States, modern folk artists carve and decorate sticks and canes more as an artistic expression than as utilitarian or fashionable walking canes. In Great Britain competitions are held to judge walking sticks and shepherd's crooks carved by amateur craftsmen.

Glass walking sticks were often called 'end of the day' by glass-blowers who would make them, together with other small souvenirs, when the day's main work was done.

Ethnic sticks and staves from Africa and the southern Pacific are generally made for the tourist trade today. Genuine old ones are hard to find, but even the modern ones make attractive souvenirs.

Because so many different materials were used, not only for the handle, but also for the shaft, today's collector has a tremendous choice should he choose to specialise and make his collection unique and original.

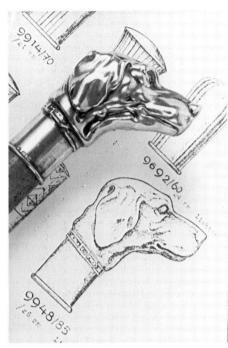

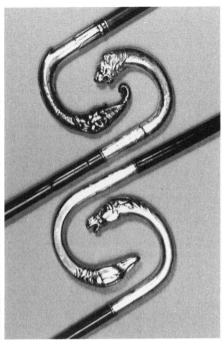

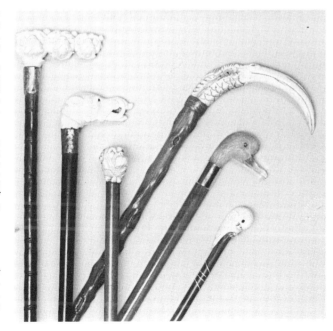

Above left: *Silver handles were manufactured by all the leading silverware factories, mainly in Great Britain and Germany. The factory of A. Moerhle in Germany still issues this dog model using the old moulds. It is shown with the original factory drawing.*

Above right: *Crook handles came into fashion towards the end of the nineteenth century and are often adorned with animal heads or the bodies of women reclining on the handle.*

Right: *Walking sticks of the late nineteenth century and early twentieth century. The duck's head is in crystal.*

7

PORCELAIN HANDLES

When porcelain was first produced in Europe, walking sticks were in high fashion with such leaders as Augustus the Strong (1670-1733) of Saxony (where Meissen porcelain originated) and Frederick the Great. Among the very first small porcelain objects that were made in Europe were knobs for canes to replace earlier Chinese knobs. Meissen itself produced 170 different designs.

Right: *The only figurative knob known from the Chelsea porcelain factory. It is attributed to Joseph Willems.*

Below: *Handle in the form of a veiled woman, issued by the KPM manufactory in Berlin by the thousands. The first model dates back to the foundation of the company in 1751. It continued to be issued throughout the nineteenth century, painted with or without the veil, and with or without the scenes by Watteau on the top. Several smaller manufacturers in Saxony copied this model in the later nineteenth century.*

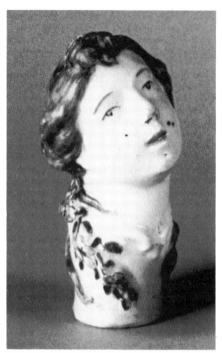

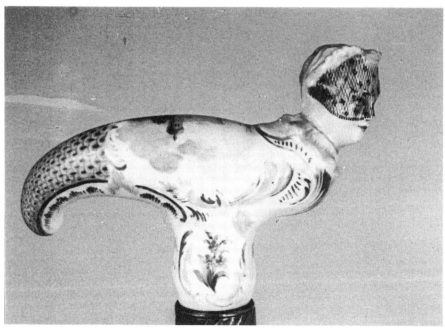

8

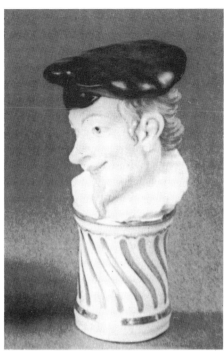

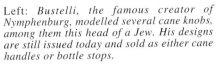

Left: *Bustelli, the famous creator of Nymphenburg, modelled several cane knobs, among them this head of a Jew. His designs are still issued today and sold as either cane handles or bottle stops.*

Below left: *Like many other souvenirs sold for the golden jubilee of Queen Victoria, this knob bears her portrait, and on the reverse side the date 1837. This does not mean that the cane belonged to her.*

Below: *Various handles and knobs typical of the nineteenth century. The one fourth from the bottom is Wedgwood.*

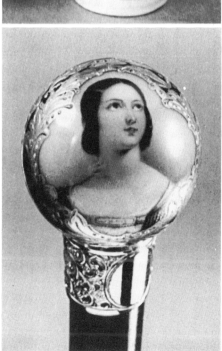

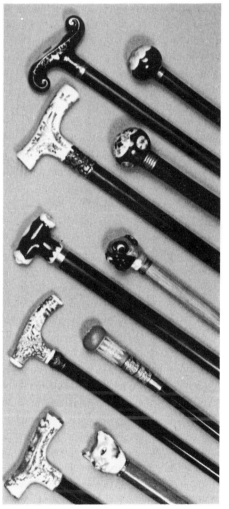

They were amongst the finest, but all the European porcelain manufacturers created knobs and handles for canes by the thousands. Today early eighteenth-century items are hard to come by, but they can easily be seen in museum porcelain collections.

In the nineteenth century many models based on earlier moulds continued to be

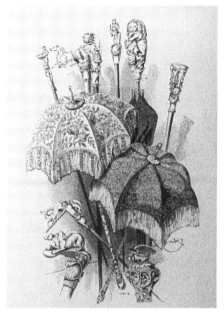

Right: *Walking sticks, umbrellas and parasols were presented for exhibition on such occasions as the Great Exhibition in Hyde Park, London, in 1851. These were from W. and J. Sangster, 140 Regent Street, London.*

Below left: *Erotic handles were quite popular at a time of strict morality. Some were more risqué than the nude women shown here, but the subject was always discreetly hidden. What is done nowadays is more pornographic than erotic.*

Below right: *Nineteenth-century walking sticks: a woman's face in Berlin metal; a figurine of Napoleon which pops out from the ivory knob; a bronze skull; a gold knob signed Valentin Morel; a bronze Leda that is a miniature version of a Pradier sculpture.*

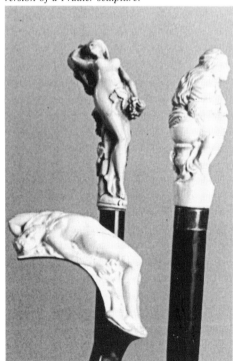

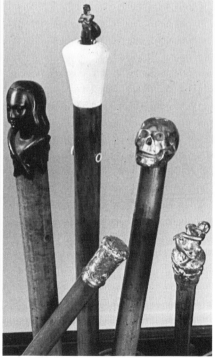

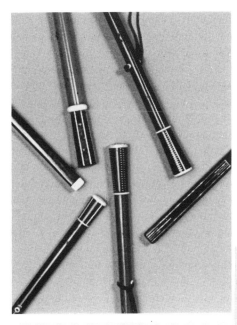

produced. As a result, normally only the quality of the decoration permits accurate attribution. It was also fashionable, towards the end of the nineteenth century, to decorate parasols and umbrellas with porcelain handles. Today one often finds these handles with very small diameters. Their size is out of proportion with the shaft of a walking stick.

Left: *Typical Art Deco walking sticks, very elegant in their sobriety.*

Below left: *Fabergé created hundreds of handles for walking sticks, parasols and crops. Some of them represent various small animals. (Photograph: Christie's, Geneva, May 1979.)*

Below: *Religious carvings are found mainly in folk art walking sticks.*

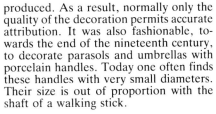

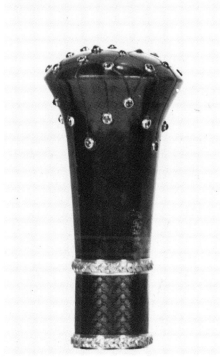

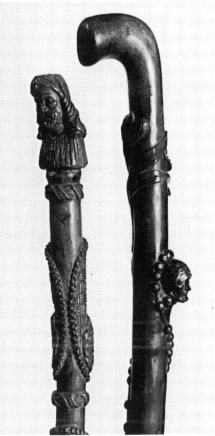

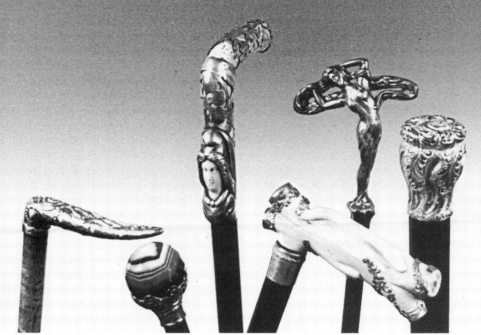

American walking sticks. (Left to right) Two models by Tiffany. An ivory and silver head of Marianne, the French emblem, covered by a liberty cap. This handle, dated 1886, was issued to commemorate the arrival of the Statue of Liberty in New York. An ivory handle with silver trimmings, a typical American handle. An Art Nouveau handle and a gold knob signed Tiffany.

Glass canes, often called 'end of the day' as, after they had finished their main work, the glassblowers created various whimsies that they would give away or sell on their own behalf. Therefore there are no records of these canes, and it is practically impossible either to date them or to certify their origin.

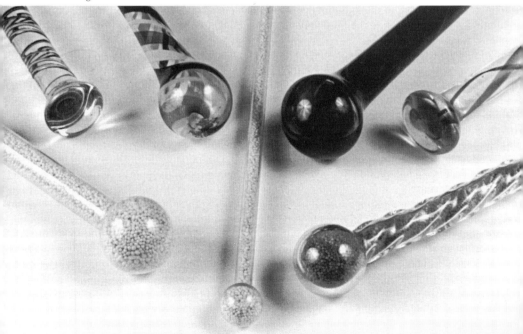

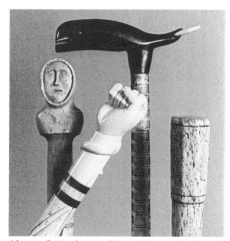

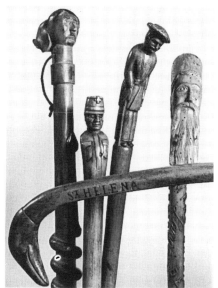

Above: *Scrimshaw walking sticks can be found in great number in the main whaling museums of the United States.*

Above right: *Prisoners' walking sticks, whittled away in captivity. (Back, from left) A head of Hitler, with the head of a pig on the reverse side; a Swiss soldier, probably carved by a French internee during the Franco-Prussian War (1870); an officer of the Indian wars; a First World War stick, with the names of all the battles fought carved along the shaft. (Front) A stick carved by a Boer prisoner interned on St Helena.*

Below: *Good examples of folk art from various countries.*

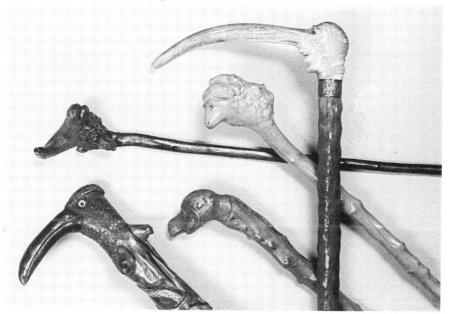

ETHNIC STICKS

Books on African or South Pacific art all mention sticks or staffs of some kind, usually covered with symbolic decoration and created for a specific task. These objects played an important part in more primitive civilisations — something which is often forgotten in western culture.

Sticks from these regions can be divided into three groups. Firstly, there are the original sticks which had very definite tribal uses. Secondly came the age of colonisation and the arrival of European men who wore canes. They, in turn, commissioned local craftsmen to make walking sticks for them, usually in the artistic style of local tribes. Thirdly, because tourism flourishes in these countries today, walking sticks are being made by the thousands preserving the symbolic styling handed down from preceding generations. This kind of walking stick is easy to find.

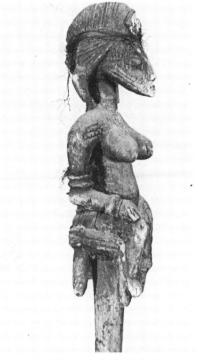

Right: A Senufo ceremonial staff from the Ivory Coast.

Below: A group of sticks from Polynesia. Every one has its own symbol and meaning.

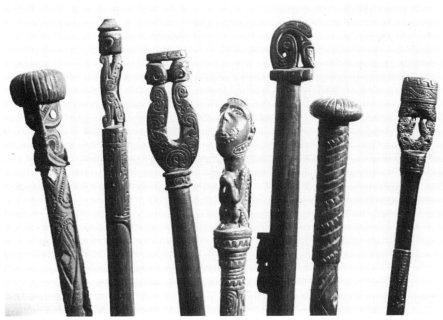

14

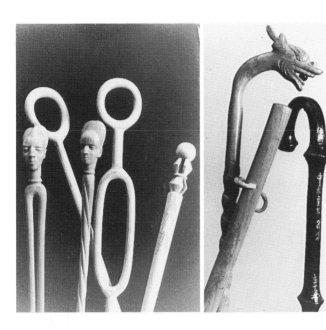

Far left: *Walking sticks from Rwanda of modern concept, but which keep the symbols of male and female that are found in other objects from the region.*

Left: *Three sticks from the Far East. (Top) A Chinese dragon: with each step the ball continues to turn, thus bringing happiness to the owner. (Centre) A simple Japanese stick used for climbing Mount Fuji. At each station a sign is painted. (Right) A black walking stick for pilgrims to the sanctuary of Datsu, Sichuan province, China.*

Below: *Souvenir walking sticks such as one can bring back from Guernsey, China, Hungary, Thailand, and various resorts in the Alps with small metal badges to be nailed on the cane. In India, inlaid sticks can be found. The two to the right come from Africa.*

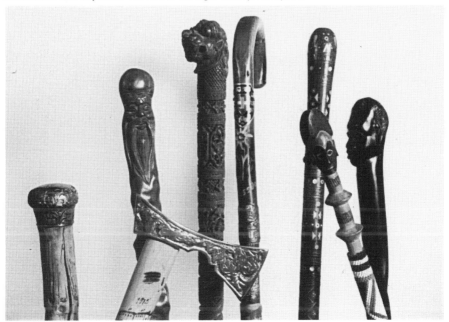

15

VARIOUS MATERIALS

At the beginning of the nineteenth century a gentleman's clothing became more and more sober and conservative. There was not much scope for originality. The band of silk, the flourish of lace and the flowing cape now belonged to an earlier age. A gentleman had little opportunity to bring fantasy to his style, manner and bearing. Even his jewellery, while it could be expensive, was limited to a watch, cuff links, gold chain and evening studs. But his walking stick was his opportunity to show his personality, his wealth, his social position, his originality. The material from which the shaft was made varied greatly. Some of the more unusual are shark spine, a ray's stinger mounted on a metal rod, hippopotamus hide, various types of horn (although rhinoceros was the most sought after), wooden shafts covered with tortoiseshell (solid tortoiseshell is quite rare), and snakeskin of many types sewn on to a fine shaft. The Victorian years produced probably the greatest assortment of any particular time.

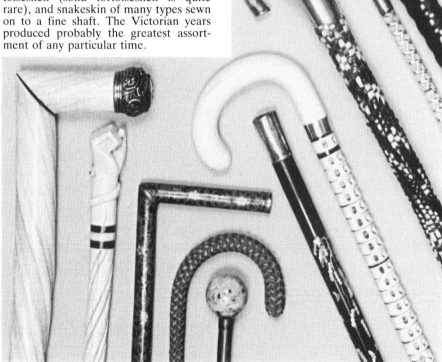

Sticks of various materials: (clockwise from top) snakeskin, natural horn, snake spine, porcupine quills, shark vertebrae, inlaid mother-of-pearl, hard stone knob, woven cord, Chinese cloisonné, scrimshaw cane, narwhal tusk.

16

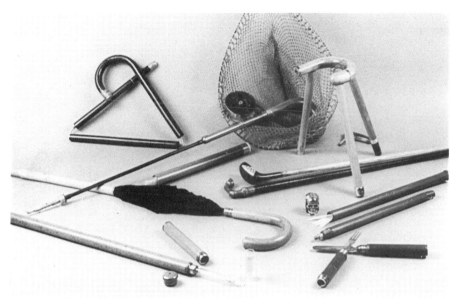

Country walking sticks with various uses: to hang one's coat on a branch; to use as a fishing rod; a net to land fish; a little stool to sit by the river; a wooden golf club and a riding whip (both are the natural length of a cane); a knife and fork for a picnic, or a little shot of brandy in the stick; an umbrella.

GADGET STICKS

The term 'gadget stick' is a new one which is applied to those walking sticks which had a dual purpose. Although approximately two thousand patents were issued for canes of this type, at no time did the words 'gadget stick' appear, and the usage is therefore strictly modern.

A distinction should be made between different kinds of gadget canes. They can be subdivided into those which contain a place in which to hide something; those with some other, purely functional alternative use, such as the capability of being converted into a seat, a music stand or a hammer; and those which represent the rank, function or profession of the owner. In certain cases the shape changes with time, as with the batons of the orchestral conductor and the field marshal.

Gadget sticks can also be divided into four main categories depending on their usage: for serious walking; for city use

(and therefore more elegant); as an emblem or tool for various professions; and as a weapon.

COUNTRY WALKING STICKS

Long after canes went out of fashion the walking stick continued to be used by many people who liked to walk in the country. In addition to providing support, it could be used to pick at ice, to test the ground, to help in ascent or descent. The handles could hide collapsible cups to be used at a mountain stream or spring, they could hold a knife and fork for picnicking, or perhaps a little flask of whisky. (A silver tippling cane was issued to commemorate the wedding of the Prince of Wales and Lady Diana Spencer in July 1981.) A compass in the handle was an obvious aid to the country walker. Other canes were devoted to pastimes such as fishing, golf, riding, butterfly catching and hunting. The gun cane was much used by poachers.

17

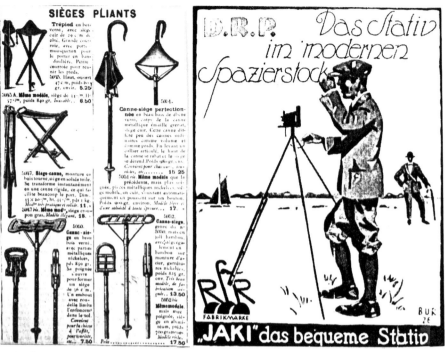

Left: *Shooting sticks were made in all shapes, and with from one to four legs. They are among the only gadget sticks still manufactured and used in modern times.*

Right: *A cane that makes a camera tripod. Tripods were used in the days when still cameras were quite heavy and had a relatively slow-speed shutter.*

Below left and right: *A patent for a bicycle in a cane! As absurd as it may seem, this patent was filed in England in 1892. 132 drawings were needed to show how to assemble it, combining the walking stick and the contents of a small bag.*

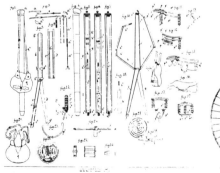
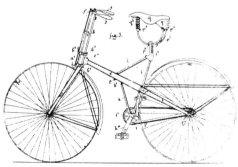

CITY WALKING STICKS

The use of a walking stick by the elegant ladies and gentlemen of the period reflected the habits and manners of the day. Pipe and chewing tobacco and snuff were often hidden in the handles as well as in the shafts, as were cigars and cigarettes, together with matches and lighters. Hollow shafts were ideal places for hiding drugs, legal or otherwise, together with the accessories needed for their use.

Before wristwatches became fashionable, the handle of a walking stick was a good place to have a watch. Optical and scientific instruments of all kinds were also incorporated into canes: spyglasses, opera glasses, binoculars, telescopes, periscopes, magnifying glasses, compasses, spectacles, microscopes, barometers and thermometers. Numerous patents have been filed for concealed cameras in cane handles — no doubt used for espionage! Hidden camera tripods were much in demand.

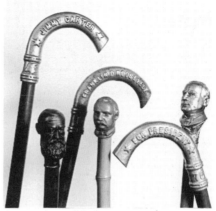

Among the political canes are the numerous sticks issued at every presidential election in the United States. Carrying a walking stick with the image of one's favoured candidate was one way to show party affiliation.

Various gadget sticks: (from left) a flashlight (these were also manufactured during the Second World War for use during blackouts); a snuffbox in a wooden shoe; a leather purse on the side to contain small change or a handkerchief; an automaton — a skull which opens its mouth; handy opera glasses which could be used discreetly; a watch; a cigarette holder in ivory; an ear trumpet which helped the deaf; a spyglass; a tobacco pipe; a religious relic; a candle with matches hidden in the ferrule; a spittoon, based on an American patent.

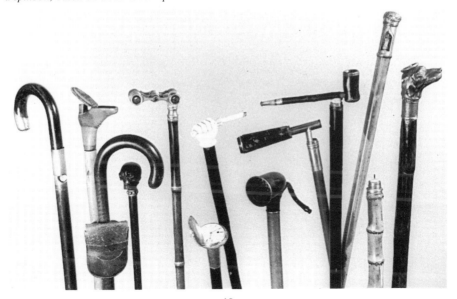

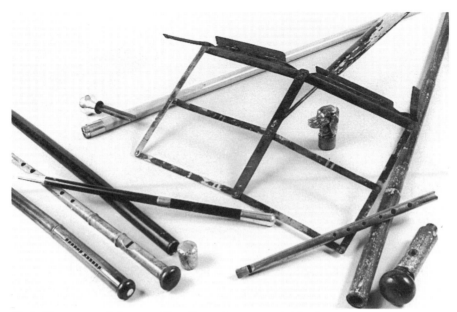

Musical instruments. Before portable radios and cassettes, a hidden flute or harmonica allowed one to have music when taking a stroll. (Clockwise from top left) A tuning fork; a music stand; a brass flageolet; a conductor's baton hidden in the shaft; a transverse metal flute; a harmonica.

Especially fine workmanship could be found in musical canes. They were real instruments. One can find beautifully made violin canes as well as canes containing guitars, zithers, bow cases, flutes of all sorts, clarinets, oboes, chanter's canes (to practise bagpipe playing), various trumpets, harmonicas, ocarinas, music stands and, perhaps not surprisingly, hidden in the shaft, tools for the piano tuner.

Ingenuity knew no bounds and fashionable ladies and gentlemen of the nineteenth century incorporated virtually every useful object into a cane or its handle, including candles, flashlights, pens and pencils, coin holders, maps, assorted games and, for the ladies, powder boxes, pillboxes, perfume bottles, atomisers, sewing kits, fans and that Victorian necessity smelling salts!

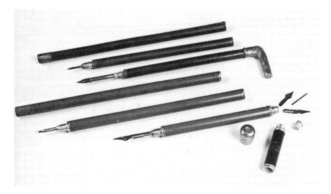

A pen and pencil holder combined to form the shaft with or without an inkstand and a reserve of pens or leads. This kind of gadget stick is often found as they were made as souvenirs for the tourists of the early twentieth century.

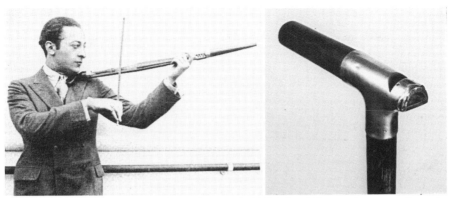

Above left: *Jascha Heifetz playing his violin cane in 1925. The violin cane is very much sought after by collectors but is a rarity.*

Above right: *Whistles were used to hail cabs.*

Below: *City walking sticks: (clockwise from the top) a glove stick to hold one's glove while kissing a lady's hand; a powder box for a lady (women 'wore' canes at different periods); a fan; a purse cane to have coins handy for giving a tip; a pillbox; a domino game; cigars (in the shaft), matches and cigar cutter (in the handle); and a locket in an ivory handle.*

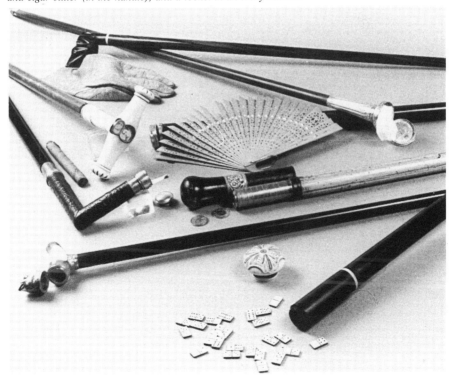

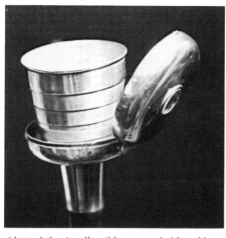 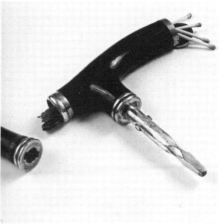

Above left: *A collapsible cup probably sold at a spa.*

Above right: *Key for a hackney carriage or railway train compartment. For security reasons the doors did not have exterior handles. This model combines a matchbox and a container for chewing tobacco.*

Below left: *A bailiff of the seventeenth century, holding his cane with a heavy round handle.*

Below right: *Canes containing ceremonial Freemason's swords. Some had scabbards, others just fitted into the shaft. The hand guards, carried separately, are missing.*

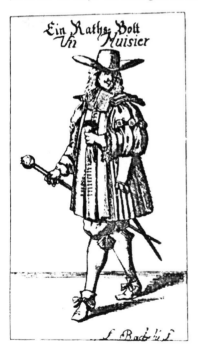 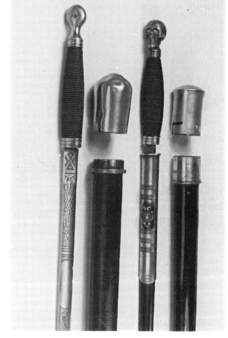

PROFESSIONAL WALKING STICKS

This category of walking stick serves to represent a trade or legal office, often with symbols pertaining to law, order and justice. Staves were adopted early on by European trade guilds to display at re-unions and parades. Perhaps the most important guild using canes was the French *compagnonage*, consisting mainly of the building trades. Each of their canes bears the emblem of a particular trade. The Knights Templar had their special walking stick, and so did the Freemasons.

Sticks have been used by civil governments and in some cases these have evolved into sceptres, magistrate's batons or even maces. The police have used staves and sticks which have latterly become truncheons and tipstaves.

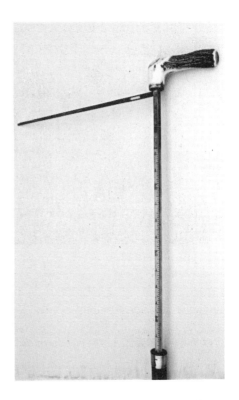

Right: *A horse-measuring walking stick still used today when buying a horse. The horizontal arm has a water level. The same principle was used for cattle and dogs. Even undertakers used this system to take measurements discreetly for the custom-made coffin. The vertical rod is then double, to measure a length of 2 metres.*

Below: *Assorted flashlights using batteries. Apart from candles in walking sticks, various fuels were used for lights in canes: oil, kerosene, acetylene, petrol and compressed gas.*

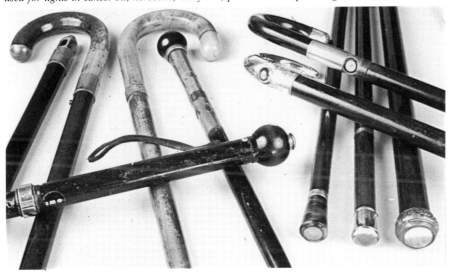

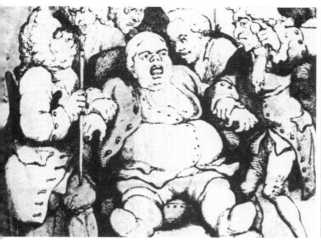

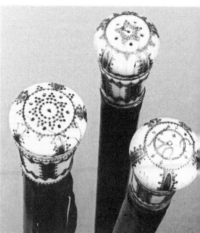

Above: *English pomanders (right) used by eighteenth- and nineteenth-century doctors to ward off epidemics and deadly fevers. An English engraving (left) caricatures the physician holding his cane below his nose. German doctors wore canes with ivory handles on which the snake of Aesculapius is carved. American doctors wore gold-headed canes.*

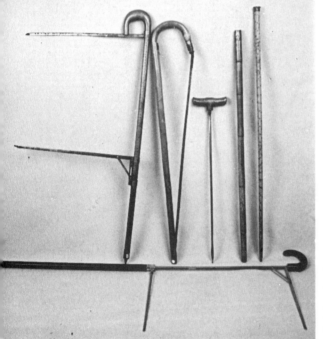

Left: *Various tools and measuring sticks: a stick to measure stacks of wood, a saw, a gimlet for probing trees, a beer-barrel measurer and a cattle measurer to measure the height, width and length of an animal in order to estimate its weight.*

Other professional sticks are those which served to contain the tools of the trade for doctors, wine traders, botanists and others. Handles shaped as hammers and hatchets were used by various trades. Measuring sticks are among the most usual instruments to be incorporated and the horse-measuring stick is still widely used. Geometers, shoemakers and tailors hid their measuring sticks in the shaft of their canes.

24

Knobsticks in the shape of heavy bronze heads.

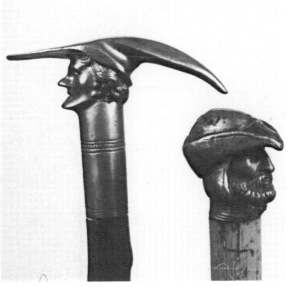

EDGED WEAPONS

Walking sticks were an ideal place to conceal weapons of various sorts. Today, in most countries, it is illegal to carry a concealed weapon, including a sword stick. However, a sturdy walking stick can be a useful defensive weapon when used properly. If the shaft is supple and the knob heavy enough, perhaps in the shape of a bronze figure for instance, much damage can be wrought. It was not uncommon to slip a rubber or metal life preserver or flails into the shaft of a walking stick.

Concealing a blade in the shaft of a cane dates back at least to the time of

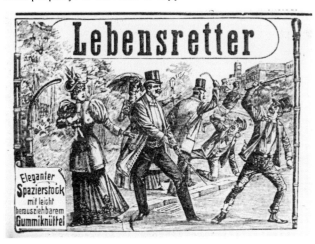

A German advertisement for life preservers.

25

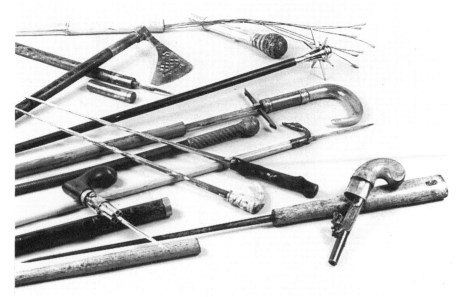

Above: *Walking sticks with concealed weapons: (clockwise from top left) a stiletto-hatchet cane; flails sunk into the shaft and covered by the handle; a life preserver with articulated spikes which fold into the handle; a Toledo blade with a hand guard; a leather knobstick; a stiletto one snaps out of the stick; two sword sticks; a flintlock pistol combined with a sword stick; a pepperbox combined with a small dagger.*

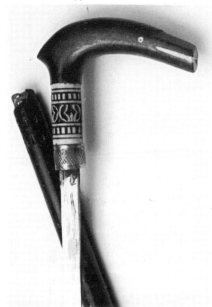

Tutankhamun (1334-25 BC), because sword sticks were found in his tomb, and possibly much earlier. During the middle ages kings and princes had blades concealed in their sticks, as did pilgrims and travellers, who would not dare to venture out on the roads without some sort of weapon for defence. These concealed blades came in all sorts of shapes and lengths. However, the most important feature was that a sword stick should not attract attention. It is quite rare to find a beautiful blade inside a top-quality shaft with an attractive or precious handle. Some canes contained vicious stilettos which snapped out of the handle. Most dangerous of all were canes with razor blades which protruded from the shaft. Anyone who attacked the holder of such an instrument would certainly regret it.

Left: *An Indian sword stick manufactured by the thousand in the 1980s and found mainly in flea markets.*

26

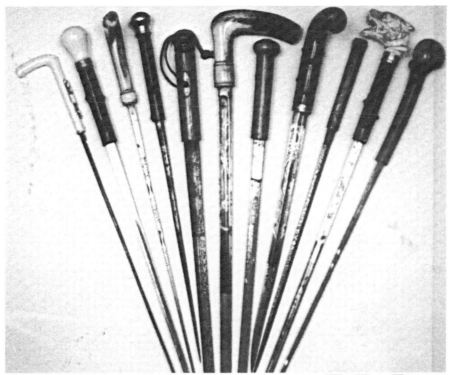

Above: *Various blades of sword sticks. Blades are often
sword blades which have been adapted to canes.*

Sword sticks can be unique and many
collectors specialise in them. Whether the
sword is signed or not, it should have a
good flexible blade and not just a piece
of metal which has been sharpened at the
end. A blade must be supple to enter with
ease into an opponent's body and cause
injury, without being stopped by a rib.

Below and right: *Deterrent spikes or razor blades emerge
when the handle and shaft are counter-twisted.*

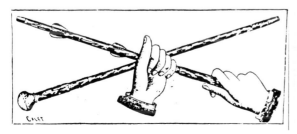

FIREARMS

When the wheel-lock gun was invented and the mechanism could be miniaturised it began to be fitted into walking sticks. Sixteenth-century pistols were often combined with a blade or a hatchet (which served as the handle). The flintlock followed and it too was quickly incorporated into walking sticks. Today these items are primarily museum pieces. In 1807, with the invention of the percussion system, the hammer could remain on the exterior of the shaft, which in turn was the barrel of the gun. To disguise it further, the whole cane was often covered in leather or veneered wood.

When cartridge cases first appeared in the middle of the nineteenth century, gun canes were mass-produced in many countries, and when the breech-loading system was invented this mass production was expanded.

Gun sticks have always been difficult to use as a defensive weapon because of their length. Pistols were therefore incor-

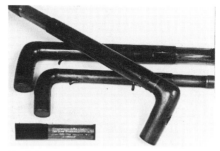

English gun canes of various calibres. These are among the few models to have a safety catch on the side. The name of the retailer often appears on the outside of the cartridge chamber.

porated into the handles, the barrel being tucked away in the shaft. These were followed by revolvers, or rather pepperboxes (in which six barrels rotate in front of the hammer, as opposed to the revolver in which the cartridges are brought in

Left: *Percussion pistols that fit into walking sticks. The handle in the shape of a duck's head has a metal bar that fits on the grip to form the butt. For the two others, the butt is carried separately.*

Right: *Underhammer percussion gun canes, the right one marked 'Day's patent'. Underhammer percussions were meant to keep the percussion cap and the gunpowder in the vent dry when it rained.*

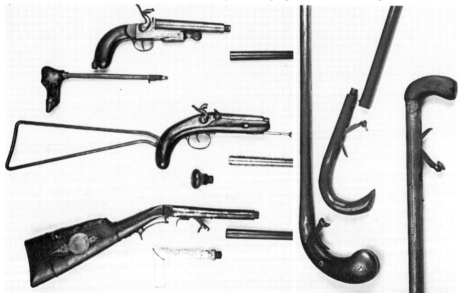

28

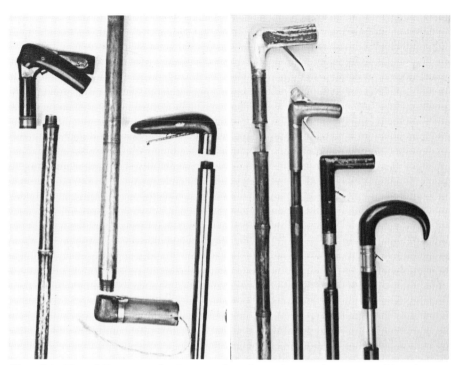

Above left: *Three different cartridge firearms, the right one having a heavy-grooved barrel.*

Above right: *Four different breech-loading firearms, the right-hand one being the type most often found.*

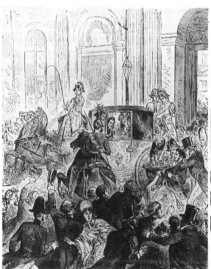

Left: *In 1836 a gun cane was used in an attempt to assassinate the French king, Louis-Philippe.*

Below: *German 'Triumph' gun canes with a long lever to cock the mechanism and expose the trigger.*

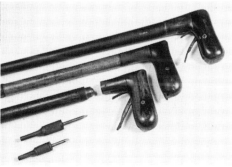

29

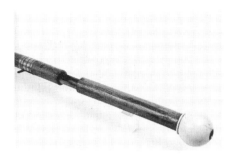

Above: *A French gun cane by Dumonthier in which the system was turned around to shoot through the handle.*

front of the single barrel). Soon the standard six-shot gun was not sufficient and machine-guns which could hold up to forty cartridges were disguised as walking sticks.

The air gun was another hunting weapon and it was ideal for poachers. Real air guns are silent and because of this were considered very dangerous. When Napoleon campaigned in Austria in 1809, anyone found in possession of an air gun was immediately executed. Once again, a walking stick was an ideal place of concealment for such a deadly weapon.

Below left: *Two American Remington gun canes with their characteristic dog head.*

Below right: *The French 'Etoile' model which was manufactured by the thousands in various calibres.*

Bottom right: *A gun cane manufactured in the 1980s. The handle is of brass and the ferrule can be used as a short dagger.*

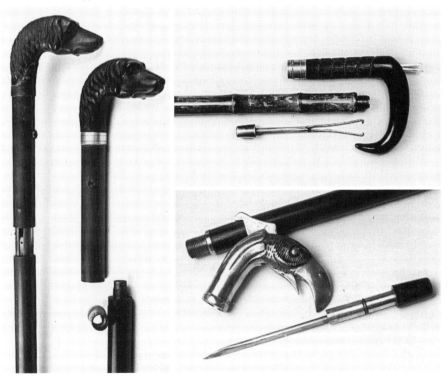

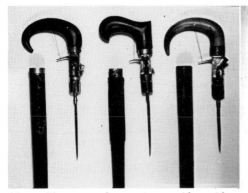

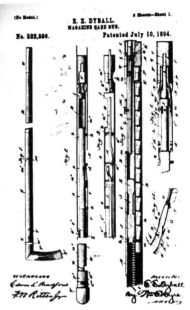

Above: *Three pepperboxes using cartridges with the three various firing devices: rim-fire, pin-fire and centre-fire. Modern cartridges should never be used on such weapons, as the powder is nowadays much stronger than at the beginning of the twentieth century.*

Right: *Dyball's patent for a 'magazine cane gun' which allowed near to thirty .22 calibre cartridges to be fitted in the shaft.*

FURTHER READING

Boothroyd, A. E. *Fascinating Walking Sticks*. White Lion Publishers, 1973.

Burcher, William, J. *The Romance behind Walking Canes*. Dorrance, Philadelphia, 1945.

Coradeschi, Sergio, and Lamberti, Alfredo. *Bastoni*. Mandadori, Milan, 1986. In Italian.

Dike, Catherine. *Cane Curiosa, from Gun to Gadget*. Les Editions de l'Amateur, Paris, and C. Dike, Geneva, 1983.

Dike, Catherine. *Canes in the United States, Illustrated Mementoes of American History, 1607-1953*. Cane Curiosa Press, Ladue, Missouri 63124, 1994.

Dike, Catherine. *Les Cannes à Systéme, un Monde Fabuleux et Méconnu*. Les Editions de l'Amateur, Paris, and C. Dike, Geneva, 1982 and 1985. In French.

Dike, Catherine. 'Silver and Gold Handles in the United States', *Silver Magazine*, Whittier, California 90609, July-September and November, 1987.

Dike, Catherine. 'What Canes are You Buying?', *The Cane Collector's Chronicle*, 2515 Fourth Avenue, Seattle Washington 98121, volume 6, number 4, 1995.

Dike, Catherine, and Bezzaz, G. *La Canne Objet d'Art*. Les Editions de l'Amateur, Paris, and C. Dike, Geneva, 1988. In French.

Douglas, John Murchie. *Blackthorn: Love and Art of Making Walking Sticks*. Alloway Publishing, 1984.

Faveton, Pierre. *Les Cannes*. Ch Massin, Paris, 1988. In French.

Fossel, Theo. *Walking and Working Sticks*. Theo Fossel, 1986. On carving walking sticks.

Girard, Sylvie. *Cannes et Parapluies et Leurs Anecdotes*. MA Editions, Paris, 1986. In French.

Grant, David, and Hart, Edward. *Shepherd's Crooks and Walking Sticks*. Mini-Books, 1972. On the carving of sticks.

Hassan, A. *Stöcke und Stäbe im Pharaonischen Aegypten.* Münchner Aegyptologische Studien, number 33, Munich, 1976. In German.

Kentucky Art and Craft Foundation and Hackley, Larry. *Historical and Contemporary Kentucky Canes.* Louisville, Kentucky, 1988.

Klever, Ulrich. *Stöcke.* W. Heyne Verlag, Munich, 1980. In German.

Klever, Ulrich. *Spazierstoöcke.* Callwey, Munich, 1984. In German.

Meyer, George H., and White, Kay. *American Folk Art Canes: Personal Sculpture.* Sandringham Press, Bloomfield Hills, Michigan 48304, 1992.

Polonec, Andrej. *Tvarované a Zdobené Palice.* Vydavatel'stvo Osveta, Martin, CS, 1977. On Slovak folk-art sticks. In Slovak with a very short résumé in English, German and Russian.

Real, Antoine. *The Story of the Stick in All Ages and Lands.* Translation by F. Fernand-Michel. J. W. Bouton, New York, 1875.

Snyder, Jeffrey B. *Canes from the Seventeenth to the Twentieth Century.* Schiffer Publishing, Atglen, Pennsylvania 19310, 1993.

Stein, Kurt. *Canes and Walking Sticks.* Liberty Caps Books, Pennsylvania, 1974.

Untersteiner, Eva. *Der Stock — Bürdezeichen, Würdeseichen.* Museum für Medizin, Dürnhof, Austria, 1985. In German.

PLACES TO VISIT

Many museums have collections of walking sticks, of greater or lesser importance, but they are nearly always stored in their reserves. Canes are considered a very minor dress accessory and will be used as props in the costume department, which usually receives the nondescript walking sticks. The departments covering archaeology, ethnography, medieval art, ivory, porcelain, glass, silver, jewellery, weapons, scientific and musical instruments, watches, et cetera, will keep the sticks appropriate to them. It takes a long time to go through all the various departments of a large museum. Porcelain departments show cane handles and knobs, so one can find some in important collections, such as at the Victoria and Albert Museum in London. Departments on folk art and ethnography might also present one or two interesting pieces.

In the United States historical societies often have numerous canes which they will show on request.

The following museums have at least ten walking sticks on display:

GREAT BRITAIN
Birmingham Museum and Art Gallery, Chamberlain Square, Birmingham, West Midlands B3 3DH. Telephone: 0121-235 2834. The Pinto Collection.

DENMARK
Rosenborg Slot, 4A Oster Voldgade, Copenhagen K.

EGYPT
Egyptian National Museum, Midan-el Tahrir, Kasr el-Nil, Cairo.

FRANCE
Musée des Arts Décoratifs, Pavillon de Marsan, 107-9 Rue de Rivoli, 75001 Paris.

GERMANY
Grünes Gewölbe, Albertinum, Georg Treu Platz, 801 Dresden.

SPAIN
Museo Federico Marés, Calle Condes de Barcelona 8, Barcelona.